REMEDIES FOR YEAST INFECTION

A path and strategy on how to be free out from and live happily.

Dr. Thomas Grey

Table of contents

INTRODUCTION
   The button line is here
CHAPTER ONE
   Understanding Yeast Infections
CHAPTER TWO
   Medical Approaches
CHAPTER THREE
   Natural Remedies
CHAPTER FOUR
   Home remedies
CHAPTER FIVE
   Home remedies that don't treat yeast infections
CHAPTER SIX
   Lifestyle Changes
CHAPTER SEVEN
   Preventive Measures
CHAPTER EIGHT
   When to See a Doctor
Conclusion
Reference page
   Disclaimer

INTRODUCTION

The button line is here

Yeast infections, caused by the overgrowth of Candida, can be uncomfortable and disrupt daily life. This guide explores various remedies, ranging from medical interventions to natural and lifestyle approaches. Understanding the causes and symptoms is crucial for effective management, and this guide aims to provide insights into both conventional and alternative methods to alleviate and prevent yeast infections. It is essential to consult with healthcare professionals for personalized advice and treatment.

CHAPTER ONE

Understanding Yeast Infections

Yeast infections, predominantly caused by the Candida fungus, occur when there's an imbalance in the body's natural flora. Candida is a type of yeast normally present in small amounts, but factors such as antibiotic use, hormonal changes, or a weakened immune system can lead to overgrowth. This guide delves into the mechanisms behind yeast infections, explaining their common symptoms and shedding light on how various factors contribute to their occurrence. A comprehensive understanding of yeast infections is essential for choosing effective remedies and preventive measures.

Typical signs of a yeast infection consist of:

- Burning and itching in the vagina and vulva
- unpleasant urination
-The vulva's swelling
-The vulva's redness
-heavy, white discharge

Obtaining an accurate diagnosis from a physician is the best line of action before attempting any home cures for yeast infections.

It's advisable to visit the doctor as soon as you start experiencing symptoms. Identifying the main causes of the yeast infection, such as illnesses resulting from weakened immune systems, is another benefit of diagnosis.

Common Causes and Symptoms

1. *Causes:*

- Antibiotic Use: Disrupts the balance of bacteria, allowing yeast to overgrow.
- Hormonal Changes: Fluctuations, as in pregnancy or during the menstrual cycle, can trigger infections.
- Weak Immune System: Compromised immunity increases susceptibility.
- Diabetes: Elevated blood sugar levels create an environment conducive to yeast overgrowth.
- Tight Clothing: Constrictive wear can create a warm, moist environment ideal for yeast.

2. ***Symptoms***:
- Itching and Irritation
- Redness and Swelling

- Unusual Discharge
- Burning Sensation
- Pain during Urination or Intercourse

Understanding these causes and symptoms is crucial for identifying and addressing yeast infections promptly.

CHAPTER TWO

Medical Approaches

1. ***Antifungal Medications***:
   - Prescription oral antifungals like fluconazole.
   - Topical antifungal creams for localized treatment.
2. ***Prescription Treatments:***
   - Stronger medications prescribed by healthcare professionals for severe cases.
3. ***Over-the-Counter Options:***
   - Antifungal creams, ointments, and suppositories available without a prescription.

Medical interventions are effective in treating yeast infections and are often recommended for swift relief. However, consulting with a healthcare provider is crucial to determine the most suitable option based on the severity of the infection.

Antifungal Medications

Antifungal medications are designed to combat yeast infections by inhibiting the growth of Candida. Two primary types are commonly used:

1. **Prescription Oral Antifungals**:
    - Examples include fluconazole (Diflucan).
    - Effective for systemic infections and cases of recurrent yeast infections.
2. **Topical Antifungal Creams**:

- Clotrimazole, miconazole, and terbinafine are common choices.
- Applied directly to affected areas for localized treatment.

It's essential to follow prescribed dosages and complete the full course of medication. Consultation with a healthcare professional helps determine the most suitable antifungal treatment based on individual circumstances.

Prescription Treatments

For more severe or persistent yeast infections, healthcare professionals may recommend stronger prescription treatments:

1. *Fluconazole (Diflucan):*
   - An oral antifungal medication.

- Effective for systemic yeast infections and cases of recurrent or resistant infections.

2. ***Itraconazole (Sporanox):***
   - Another oral antifungal option.
   - Used in cases where fluconazole may be less effective.

3. ***Topical Prescription*** Medications:
   - Creams or ointments with higher concentrations of antifungal agents.
   - Applied directly to affected areas under the guidance of a healthcare provider.

Prescription treatments are tailored to the specific needs and severity of the yeast infection, emphasizing the importance of consulting with a healthcare professional for appropriate diagnosis and treatment.

Over-the-Counter Options

For milder cases of yeast infections, over-the-counter (OTC) options are available without a prescription:

1. ***Antifungal Creams:***
    - Common ingredients include clotrimazole (Lotrimin), miconazole (Monistat), and tioconazole.
    - Applied externally to alleviate symptoms and combat yeast overgrowth.
2. ***Antifungal Suppositories:***
    - Inserts containing antifungal agents like clotrimazole or miconazole.
    - Designed for internal use to address infections from within.

3. ***Oral Antifungal Medications***:
   - Some oral antifungal medications may be available without a prescription.
   - Follow package instructions and use as directed.

While OTC options can be effective for certain cases, it's crucial to read instructions carefully and seek professional advice if symptoms persist or worsen. Consulting a healthcare provider ensures appropriate treatment and addresses individual health considerations.

CHAPTER THREE

Natural Remedies

1. ***Probiotics:***
   - Introduction of beneficial bacteria to restore microbial balance.
   - Found in supplements or fermented foods like yogurt and kefir.
2. ***Garlic:***
   - Contains allicin, known for its antifungal properties.
   - Consumed raw, as a supplement, or incorporated into meals.
3. ***Tea Tree Oil:***
   - Exhibits antifungal and antibacterial properties.

- Diluted and applied topically; caution is advised due to its potency.

4. *Yogurt:*
  - Contains probiotics and may help restore healthy flora.
  - Applied topically or consumed to support internal balance.

While natural remedies can offer relief, it's essential to use them cautiously and in conjunction with professional advice. Consultation with a healthcare provider ensures a holistic approach to managing yeast infections.

YEAST INFECTION PREVENTED NATURALLY.

Prevention is the best medicine when it comes to yeast infections. To reduce the possibility of getting a yeast infection:One

Keep soap and douche out of your vagina.Wear breathable, loose-fitting cotton panties.

Quickly change out of your damp bathing suit or sweaty gym attire.

Avert perfumed detergents and soaps.

Frequently replace tampons and pads.

Always wipe from the front to the rear when using the loo.

Refrain from overindulging in hot tubs and really hot baths.

Reduce your intake of foods that cause yeast, such as alcohol and Sugar.

An antifungal medication is the most effective technique to treat a yeast infection.

Although there are many do-it-yourself solutions available, taking antifungal medication is the quickest (and most effective) way to treat yeast infections.

Antifungal drugs either eradicate or inhibit the development of fungi, including yeast. This can be in the form of capsule suppositories, topical lotions, or edible pills. The most commonly used ones to treat infections are fluconazole, nystatin, ciclopirox, and clotrimazole. You can purchase over-the-counter drugs such as Diflucan and Mycostatin.

A 2019 study concluded that anyone with complex or recurrent vaginal yeast infections needs to see a doctor. They can recommend a long-term course of therapy in addition to a diet rich in beneficial microorganisms.

Here are some natural treatments for yeast infections that may or may not help for those who would rather treat their infection at home.

CHAPTER FOUR

Home remedies

1. *Vinegar Baths:*

- Apple Cider Vinegar Bath:
    - Adding a cup of apple cider vinegar to a warm bath may help rebalance pH levels.
    - Soak for 15-20 minutes, ensuring proper dilution.

2. *Coconut Oil:*

- Topical Application:
    - Applying coconut oil externally may offer relief from itching and irritation.
    - Ensure the coconut oil used is pure and free from additives.

3. *Boric Acid Suppositories*:

- Antifungal Properties:
    - Suppositories with boric acid can help combat yeast infections.
    - Use under the guidance of a healthcare professional due to potential side effects.

While these home remedies are considered by some, it's essential to approach them with caution. Consultation with a healthcare provider is crucial, especially before using boric acid, to ensure safety and effectiveness in individual cases.

Yeast infection home cures

The following home treatments for yeast infections have been well researched, and there is enough proof to suggest that they can either cure the infection or at least lessen the chance that it will return:

1. Consume probiotics.

 Healthy bacteria are introduced into the vagina by certain types of probiotics, particularly Lactobacillus. As a result of the bacteria in the vagina being balanced again, this may help treat yeast infections and enhance vaginal health in general.

In a 2015 study, probiotic Lactobacillus effectively stopped the recurrence of infection in 19 women with recurrent yeast infections. One year later, an 89% cure rate was seen in those who utilised vaginal capsules containing Lactobacillus for 10 days in addition to medicine. Conversely, 70% of individuals who only took medication saw a 12-month cure rate. "It's actually when someone stops or removes the probiotics from their regimen when they will develop a yeast infection," explains Tamika Auguste, an obstetrician and gynaecologist at Medstar Washington Hospital Centre in Washington, DC. As such, several medical professionals advise against using probiotics as your only form of treatment. Rather, they might serve as more of a prophylactic precaution.

Increasing your intake of lactobacillus-rich foods like kombucha, sauerkraut, and miso is one simple method to incorporate probiotics into your diet. Enhancing vaginal health may also benefit from probiotic supplements containing at least one billion colony-forming units (CFUs).

Probiotic suppositories are capsules containing the Lactobacillus strain that are inserted directly into the vagina. These introduce the good bacteria directly into the vagina and restore its balance. It can also help treat and prevent bacterial vaginosis and recurring urinary tract infections.

2. ***Try boric acid***: Boric acid is a powdery substance with antifungal properties and probiotics like Lactobacilliales, meaning it balances the bacteria in the vagina, thereby treating yeast infections. Early evidence of boric acid's ability to treat yeast infections is promising. For example, a 2011 literature review in the Journal of Women's Health looked at 14 separate studies where the efficacy of the substance was compared to nine other antifungals like fluconazole and

terconazole. The review found that boric acid cured between 40% to 100% of patients. You can find boric acid at a grocery store, usually in the pharmacy or cleaning aisle. To treat yeast infections, place about 600mg of boric acid into suppository capsules — cone-shaped pills that dissolve in your body — that can then be inserted into the vagina. Standard treatment requires using a pill once a day before bed for seven days straight.

CHAPTER FIVE

Home remedies that don't treat yeast infections

The following natural remedies lack evidence for their effectiveness in treating yeast infections at home:

1. *Avoid garlic*: Some have suggested garlic is a good over-the-counter remedy for yeast infections. That's because allicin, a substance released when fresh garlic is crushed, has well-known antimicrobial and antibacterial properties that can damage bacterial yeasts. However, these benefits do not outweigh the risks. Auguste says she does not recommend garlic as an at-home treatment for yeast infections due to potential side effects. Placing raw garlic in your vaginal canal not only introduces a foreign object, but she says it can also cause skin in the canal to burn and become irritated. Moreover, there's limited research to suggest that garlic is more effective than other treatments. For example, a 2010 study looked at the effect of treating yeast infections with a medicinal cream filled with garlic and thyme and how it compared with a typical clotrimazole vaginal cream, an antifungal cream available over the counter or by prescription. The garlic cream was just as effective as the clotrimazole. However, the population studied was quite small, and the group using the garlic treatment reported more side effects overall. According to Auguste, "there's no proof that a clove of garlic alone will prevent or treat an infection.

2. *Be wary of tea tree oil*

Tea tree oil is often marketed as a natural.

substance to help manage acne and other skin conditions. But, there is debate as to whether it can help with yeast infections. On its own, it certainly won't cure an infection. But it could prove helpful when combined with other treatments in certain cases.

CHAPTER SIX

Lifestyle Changes

1. ***Diet Modifications:***
   - Limit Sugar Intake:
     - Reducing sugar helps create an environment less favorable for yeast.
   - Probiotic-Rich Foods:
     - Incorporate yogurt, kefir, and fermented foods to support a healthy balance of bacteria.
2. ***Clothing Choices:***
   - Cotton Underwear:
     - Allows better air circulation, minimizing moisture.
   - Loose-Fitting Clothing:

- Helps prevent a warm and damp environment conducive to yeast growth.

3. ***Personal Hygiene Tips***:
   - Avoid Harsh Soaps:
     - Use mild, fragrance-free soaps to avoid irritation.
   - Regular Showers:
     - Maintain good hygiene practices without overwashing, which can disrupt the natural flora.

Adopting these lifestyle changes alongside other remedies contributes to a comprehensive approach in preventing and managing yeast infections. Individual responses may vary, so consulting with a healthcare professional is advised for personalized guidance.

CHAPTER SEVEN

Preventive Measures

1. ***Maintaining a Healthy Diet:***
   - Balanced Nutrition:
     - Consume a diet rich in fruits, vegetables, and whole grains.
     - Limit sugar intake to help prevent conditions favorable for yeast growth.
2. ***Proper Hygiene Practices:***
   - Gentle Cleansing:
     - Use mild, fragrance-free soaps to maintain cleanliness without disrupting natural flora.

- Dry thoroughly after bathing to prevent moisture buildup.

3. ***Avoiding Triggers:***

   Avoid Harsh Products:

   - Steer clear of harsh detergents, scented products, and feminine hygiene sprays.
   - Opt for breathable, cotton underwear and clothing.

Implementing these preventive measures helps create an environment less conducive to yeast infections. Individual responses may vary, so it's advisable to consult with a healthcare professional for personalized guidance on maintaining optimal health and preventing recurring infections.

Can a yeast infection go away on its own?

For those with busy schedules or upcoming trips and exciting plans, it's not what you want to hear — but only the mildest yeast infections can be successfully treated using the at-home tools we've highlighted above. More often than not, especially if you are experiencing severe symptoms that are new to you, you'll need to call your doctor or head to an emergency clinic to confirm your diagnosis and to receive a prescription for antifungal medications.

The good news? These medications may work to resolve the yeast overgrowth, and quell subsequent symptoms, in as little as 24 hours. Most will clear up within days, and you should be able to resume normal routines soon.

You may have more success by incorporating holistic preventative measures into your routine targeted to preventing further yeast infections — like probiotics, for example. Probiotic supplements containing Lactobacillus help to relate your vagina's bacteria, especially those that contain more than 1 billion colony-forming units (CFUs), which can help stave off yeast overgrowth as well as issues like urinary tract infections.

Use tea tree oil with caution
Tea tree oil is frequently promoted as a natural remedy for acne and other skin issues. However, its ability to treat yeast infections is up for debate. It most definitely won't treat an infection on its own. However, in certain circumstances,

it might be beneficial when used with other treatments.

Does a yeast infection resolve itself?

It's not what you want to hear, but the at-home remedies we've mentioned above can only effectively treat the mildest yeast infections. This is especially true for individuals with hectic schedules, exciting travels, and plans. For the most part, you will need to contact your doctor or go to an emergency clinic in order to get your diagnosis confirmed and to get a prescription for antifungal medications, especially if you are having severe symptoms that are unfamiliar to you.

The favorable tidings? In as little as 24 hours, these drugs may be able to stop the overgrowth of yeast and all associated symptoms. Most will go away in a few days, so you should soon be able to get back to your regular schedule.

You may have more success by including holistic preventative measures into your regimen targeted to preventing further yeast infections — like probiotics, for example. Probiotic supplements with Lactobacillus aid in the relationship between the bacteria in your vagina, particularly those with more than 1 billion colony-forming units (CFUs), which can help prevent yeast overgrowth and other problems including UTIs.

How can you care for yourself at home?

Take your medicines exactly as prescribed. Call your doctor or nurse advice line if you think you are having a problem with your medicine. Ask your doctor about over-the-counter (OTC) medicines for yeast infections. If you use an OTC treatment, read and follow all instructions on the label. Don't use tampons while using a vaginal cream or suppository. The tampons can absorb the medicine. Use pads instead. Wear loose cotton clothing. Don't wear nylon or other fabric that holds body heat and moisture close to the skin. Try sleeping without underwear. Don't scratch. Relieve itching with a cold pack or a cool bath. Don't wash your vulva more than once a day. Use plain water or a mild, unscented soap. Air-dry the vulva. Change out of wet or damp clothes as soon as possible. If you are using a vaginal medicine, don't have sex until you have finished your treatment. But if you do have sex, don't depend on a latex condom or diaphragm for birth control. The oil in some vaginal medicines weakens latex. Don't douche or use powders, sprays, or perfumes in your vagina or on your vulva. These items can change the normal balance of organisms in your vagina. Symptoms Yeast infections with discharge look thick and white, like cottage cheese. Other symptoms of a vulvovaginal yeast infection include itching, burning, or irritation of the vagina or vulva, which is the tissue surrounding the vagina pain or soreness in the vagina or the vaginal opening vaginal burning with intercourse or urination a watery discharge a rash Sometimes a more complicated yeast infection may occur with more severe symptoms. Four or more infections may arise in 1 year. Doctors refer to this as recurrent vulvovaginal candidiasis

(RVVC). There may be severe redness, swelling, and itching, leading to skin fissures or sores with a complicated yeast infection. Medical conditions that can cause a complicated yeast infection or RVVC include: pregnancy unmanaged diabetes having a weakened immune system the presence of an alternate Candida fungus, as opposed to Candida albicans.

In males, a yeast infection can affect the head of the penis. Symptoms include redness, irritation, and discharge. It can also affect the skin or the mouth.

Treatment

The fastest way to get rid of a yeast infection is to contact a doctor. They can provide a timely and accurate diagnosis. They will prescribe the right treatment for the condition.

Most cases of vaginal yeast infection are mild, and the condition is not bothersome. Some people have no symptoms at all.

recommends contacting a doctor if there are symptoms such as:

-itching

-soreness

-pain

-atypical discharge

Treatment of the infection depends on whether it is complicated or uncomplicated.

A complicated yeast infection may involve

More symptoms or they may be more severe. For example, a person may experience vaginal or labial swelling. Another sign of a complication is if a person has repeated infections or if the infections occur due to a weakened immune system.

Uncomplicated yeast infection

There are two ways to treat an uncomplicated yeast infection: vaginal therapy or oral treatment.
When treating an uncomplicated yeast infection, a short course of vaginal therapy is usually sufficient.
One option is a one-time treatment of a prescription or an over-the-counter (OTC) medication, such as:
butoconazole (Gynazole-1)
clotrimazole (Gyne-Lotrimin)
miconazole (Monistat 3)
terconazole (Terazol 3)
Some of these are available to buy online, including clotrimazole, Monistat 3, and terconazole.
Because these medications are oil-based, they can weaken latex

condoms and diaphragms, potentially making them less reliable. A person can use non latex-based condoms instead. Alternatively, an oral antifungal such as fluconazole (Diflucan) can be used in one single dose.

A yeast infection might impact the penis' head in men. Redness, discomfort, and discharge are some of the symptoms. It may also have an impact on the lips or skin.

Handling.

Making a doctor's appointment is the quickest way to treat a yeast infection. They are able to offer a prompt and precise diagnosis. They will recommend the best course of action for the ailment. The majority of vaginal yeast infections are not severe, and the illness is not uncomfortable. Some folks don't even exhibit any symptoms. suggests calling a doctor if you experience any symptoms, like itching or pain, suffering and unusual discharge.

Whether an infection is difficult or not determines how it should be treated. The symptoms of a complex yeast infection could be more numerous or more severe. One could get vaginal or labial edema, for instance.
If an individual experiences recurrent infections or if their immune system is compromised, this could also indicate a potential problem.

Simple yeast infection

An oral treatment or vaginal therapy are the two options for treating an uncomplicated yeast infection.

For the treatment of a simple yeast infection, a brief course of vaginal medication is typically adequate.

A prescription or over-the-counter (OTC) medicine used as a one-time treatment is one alternative. Examples of such medications are butoconazole (Gynazole-1), clotrimazole (Gyne-Lotrimin), miconazole (Monistat 3), and terconazole (Terazol 3), Some of these, such terconazole, Monistat 3, and clotrimazole, can be purchased online.

These drugs can damage latex condoms and diaphragms, which could make them less dependable, because they are oil-based. Instead, non-latex condoms can be used.

As an alternative, a single dose of an oral antifungal such fluconazole (Diflucan) can be administered.

complicated yeast infection

Treatment for a severe yeast infection may need long-term vaginal treatments or oral formulations taken in multiple doses.

It's possible for a doctor to suggest maintenance drugs. These medications may be taken on a daily basis to stop the infection from coming back.

Using a vaginal cream, ointment, pill, or suppository for seven to fourteen days is known as long-course vaginal therapy.
Occasionally, a physician may advise against vaginal therapy in favor of two to three oral fluconazole doses.

A doctor may recommend topical steroids for a few days to assist manage symptoms while the antifungal medicine is taking effect if the patient's symptoms are severe.

It's critical to confirm if the symptoms are caused by a yeast infection before using antifungals. Antifungals may become less effective in the future when needed since abuse of them can lead to yeast resistance.

When one of the aforementioned treatment modalities is ended, maintenance drugs are started if needed. For six months, it can entail either weekly vaginal clotrimazole treatments or weekly oral fluconazole treatments.

Treatment may also be warranted if the person's sexual partner exhibits symptoms of yeast infection. The use of condoms or other barrier techniques is frequently advised by medical practitioners.

CHAPTER EIGHT

When to See a Doctor

1. ***Signs of Complications***:
   - Persistent or severe symptoms despite home remedies and over-the-counter treatments.
   - Recurrent yeast infections within a short period.
   - Unusual or worrisome changes in discharge, odor, or appearance.
2. ***Seeking Professional Advice***:
   - First-Time Infections:
     - If experiencing symptoms for the first time, consult a healthcare professional

for accurate diagnosis
and guidance.

3. ***Pregnancy:***

Pregnant individuals should
seek medical advice due to
potential risks.

4. ***Underlying Health Conditions:***
Individuals with weakened immune
systems or diabetes should consult
a doctor for tailored
recommendations.

Prompt consultation with a healthcare
provider ensures proper diagnosis and
appropriate treatment, reducing the risk
of complications and addressing specific
health considerations

Conclusion

Effectively managing and preventing
yeast infections involves a combination
of medical treatments, natural remedies,
lifestyle adjustments, and preventive
measures. Understanding the causes,
symptoms, and various available options
is crucial for informed decision-making.
While over-the-counter and home
remedies can offer relief, seeking
professional advice, especially in the
case of persistent or severe symptoms,
is paramount. Adopting a holistic
approach, including maintaining a
healthy diet and proper hygiene
practices, contributes to long-term
well-being. Individual responses may

vary, so consulting with a healthcare professional ensures tailored guidance for optimal health and the prevention of recurrent infections.

Reference page

Disclaimer

Consider this as advice: a reader is not supposed to use this as a prescription, make sure that you keep in touch with your doctor before using this as a prescription.

Hello, if you find this note helpful please I need your good reviews. Thank you as you do so.